42 tips that will make you a better runner.

by Andreas Michaelides

The information contained in this book is intended to be educational and not for diagnosis, prescription, or treatment of any health disorder whatsoever.

This book is sold with the understanding that neither the author nor publisher is engaged in rendering any medical or psychological advice. Readers should consult their physician prior to beginning a new exercise program, changing their diet, quitting smoking, or making other lifestyle changes.

The publisher and author disclaim personal liability, directly or indirectly, for the information presented within.

Although the author and publisher have prepared this manuscript with utmost care and diligence and have made every effort to ensure the accuracy and completeness of the information contained within, we assume no responsibility for errors, inaccuracies, omissions, or inconsistencies.

42 tips that will make you a better runner.

ISBN: 9789963277018
Cyprus Library.
www.cypruslibrary.gov.cy

Table of Contents

Tip number 1: Always have a training plan.

If you want to call yourself a runner, you need to be able to track changes that are happening in your fitness level. To do that, you will need to have a training program that will gradually increase your training load. Also, the difference between a jogger and a runner, among other things, is that a jogger doesn't have a training program; he or she just goes for a run without having in mind the fulfillment of specific goals.

If you want to call yourself a runner you need to set goals, like completing your first 5km race or your first 10km race, and so on.

To achieve that, apart from a tremendous self-discipline, you will need to create a training program that will contain the following:

Running training sessions, weightlifting sessions, XT (Alternative to running) sessions, rest days, and nutritional support of your training.

Make sure to make it as flexible as you can to anticipate little obstacles life throws at you.

As an example, let's say you have Track training on Monday and Weightlifting on Tuesday (Biceps and Triceps), and on Monday something happens, and you lose the Track training. It's not the end of the world; do the Weightlifting on Monday, which will obviously take less time, and do the Track repeats on Tuesday.

Another example, you can't do the long run-on Sunday because you must attend a family gathering or something similar, time-consuming event. Do the long run-on Saturday and do the Saturday activities on Sunday, or even better, switch the rest day on Sunday and do the long run on your rest day.

Improvise and adapt and you will see you will reach a point that you can do stuff out of thin air!

Tip number 2: Be a little Selfish.

As we get older and as we create a family, wife/husband and kids, and other family-oriented activities, we tend to devote most of our free time and, sometimes, all our own time to our loved ones, spouse, and children.

I used to do that too, and I think it's important to understand that both our psychological and physical health must be our highest priority. Running achieves both at the same time. It helps us deal with stress by reducing it and keeps us fit and healthy by strengthening our immune system.

When we are healthy, then we can provide more to our family members, like spouse and kids. When we are sick and depressed, we are not much help, first to ourselves and then to our family and friends.

So, it's in our best interest both individually and socially for us to be in a healthy state.

So, the next time you feel guilty that you are stealing time from doing something else with your family, remember that you need some alone quality time too and try to see the big picture; focus on the beautiful forest, not the tree. A healthy you mean a better-quality time with your family, and running will provide that for you, if you manage to put some time to practice it without feelings of regret or feeling that you are letting others down.

Tip number 3: Minimize TV watching.

Have you ever sat down and calculated how much time you spend in front of the TV daily? If you didn't, then please do it, and if you find out that you spend more than 30 minutes a day, then you need to start reducing the hours you waste watching TV gradually.

The time that you waste on TV, you can allocate it to do more meaningful and more important things for you and your family. On average, most people spend 2 to 4 hours every day watching TV, not continuously of course but nevertheless, think about it, people, 4 hours, that's 240 minutes of your time that you can use to do so much more.

I used to watch much TV in the past also; I would come from home, eat, take a shower, and then sit for hours in front of the "stupid box" watching whatever I found interesting.

Don't get me wrong, I do know that TV has its good sides too, it has some informative shows, like documentaries or other kinds of useful information, but wasting that many hours in front of it is not healthy and is not productive.

Now what I do is I watch a movie every Friday night, and if there is a documentary that I can use its information in an article of mine, on my blog or in one of my books, then it's not a waste of time but an investment in developing skills and enhancing the value of my work; it's an advantage instead of a disadvantage.

Reduce TV watching to 30 minutes per day, in fact, if you can get rid of it altogether, the better. Now I use Netflix for my viewing pleasure, it's cheap, and I can watch it whenever and wherever I want. I always watch documentaries that are about quitting smoking or weight loss or culinary situations or about running, subjects that I am intrigued and interested in, and, as I said earlier, will help me with my article and book writing.

Trust me on this, stop watching so much tv and you'll see you will have adequate time to go walking or running or do the exercise you love, more time for your family and friends. More importantly of all, you will have more time to start living your life, you and not the actors on TV.

Tip number 4: Minimize Social Media Interaction.

In the old days, at least you only had the stupid box to waste your time; now, we have the Internet and all these social media that are popping up every 3 to 6 months, asking for our attention and our precious time.

Again, the same advice, stop wasting your time on the computer, playing around with social media (Facebook likes, Twitter follows, and pin that, and share that, and so on). Do not answer to every email you receive immediately! Stop messaging everybody every 5 minutes.

Minimize your time spent online and invest that time in something more productive; something that will make you a better person either in skills or in knowledge or behavior.

So, the same thing as I asked you with TV, applies here as well; sit down and calculate how much time you spend on online social media; it's the same amount of time you always complain about not having enough to do things!

I used to be like that, spending countless hours in front of the computer monitor, watching videos, chatting, playing online computers games with "friends" all around the world, sharing, liking wasting my precious time away and not learning something useful for my future.

I don't do that anymore, though. I spend 15 minutes in the morning to have a quick look at my social media status, check my emails, and reply to the ones I think are important and meaningful, and that's it.

Then, at night, a few minutes before I go to bed, I will give my email a quick view to see if I have something important, and that's it. I minimize my internet consumption to 30 minutes tops per day.

Tip number 5: Go to bed early.

I know this is not always possible, especially when you have little humans running around the house refusing to go to sleep, but you are the parent, so act like one, don't let these little people govern your life; you are the adult; enforce some rules.

Try to go to bed as early as you can, try to catch at least 7 to 8 hours of sleep. I know some of you may be laughing right now but make the effort to get 7 to 8 hours of sleep, preferably between 9 p.m. and five a.m., this is the time we evolved to get our precious rest.

If you go early to bed, you rest; your batteries will be charged; you wake up early in the morning, and you can do more stuff, either something personal, like going for a 30-minute run around the block or making breakfast for the kids.

Sleep deprivation, as shown in studies, causes obesity and heart conditions.

Tip Number 6: Wake up early

If you go to bed early, you wake up early and, as I mentioned, you can do more stuff. Except exercising or taking care the needs of the family, you can use that time to employ some relaxing activities, like breathing techniques that will help you reduce stress and anxiety and some yoga exercises that will also help you relax and acquire physiological flexibility, which is proven in studies that enhance our immune system. A boosted and healthy immune system does not allow a common illness like the flu or other trivial illnesses to bother you, increasing, therefore, your productivity and both your work with your hobbies and with your family.

Tip number 7: Run at least 3 to 4 times per week.

When I first started running back in 2010 again, I was running everyday nonstop; in the back of my head, I had this notion that a day without running was a lost day! Now I know better, resting days, and what I mean by resting days is not run less or run with less intensity, but be a lazy for a day, do not run at all, just rest, and let your body recover and repair itself.

Now the most I run is four days a week, and I do that if I am incorporating some hill training in my schedule to make my legs stronger. Otherwise, I will run three times a week minimum.

I do three distinct exercises and after testing the FIRST program, I became a fan! THE FIRST program is a program that is perfect for everybody because it is so adaptable, and time saving, and you can see results fast.

The FIRST program is the baby of Bill Pierce, Scott Murr, and Ray Moss, and you can find it in their book entitled **_Run Less Run Faster_**, how cool is that?

The program advocates running three times a week doing, as I mentioned, three different kinds of exercises.

First Exercise is **_Track Repeats_**; this type of training will increase and optimize your speed.

The second exercise is **_Tempo Runs_**; you set a specific distance or distances, and you aim to run them with an accurate pace from start to finish. This kind of training optimizes the ability of the runner to maintain a certain tempo for a certain distance also increasing the endurance of the athlete.

The third exercise is the classical **_Long Run_** where you run on a slightly lower tempo than your race tempo, and the goal of this training is to increase your aerobic capacity and train your body to burn more body fat than glucose in the long run.

That's what I do now; on Monday, I do Track Repeats on the high school's track here in my village.

On Thursday, I do Tempo Runs and on Sunday or Saturday, depending which day I have more time, I do my Long Runs.

Track Repeats and Tempo Runs do not take me more than an hour, and Long Runs way more, depending on the week I am into my training.

This kind of training has a lot of advantages. First, you don't get injured easily since you are only running three times a week. Second, you don't get bored or get tired of running because you have at least a day off between the periods of training and so you can relax and recover for your next run. Third, it is a time saver; you don't feel like you have a second job to be able to train for a marathon or half marathon. For smaller distances like 10km or 5km, the time you spend for training every week is maybe 3 to 4 hours tops; that's nothing!

So, my advice if you are training for races from 5km until Marathon, have a look at this FIRST training program. I tested it, and it works.

Tip number 8: Strengthening exercises 2 to 3 times a week.

As I mentioned in my previous tip, when I first started running, I would run every day nonstop, without any resting days, which now I know it was a mistake, that's why I gave you tip number 7.

Another error was not to train my upper core namely abs, chest, back, arms, etc. The reason I was not doing that was because, in the back of my ignorant mind, I had this idea that I only need to have strong legs to run, that running was purely a leg's work, and any extra weight on my upper body would be a burden that would slow me down!

Even if there is a small truth in that predicament, having a strong core is the Alpha and Omega for running, and not just for running, but for every exercise you do.

If you have a weak core, then, after running for a period, those muscles get tired and at some point, they give up, they collapse, and other muscle groups are asked to do their job. When you have weak abs after serious running, if they collapse and cannot maintain the balance and the stability they offer, then the burden of their work falls on the legs and more frequently on the knees and on the ankles.

This leads, as a result, to have knee injuries, which is one of the most common injuries runners have, I.T.B. (Iliotibial Band Syndrome) injuries, and so on.

It is paramount to have a strong upper body and muscles that can support your running from the beginning until the end.

Imagine your core to be the air in your car tires. When the air in your tires is not enough, the tires do not produce the maximum, and because of the friction that is created due to the lack of it, the car needs more energy to burn to go forward.

You need to have your muscles pump up enough to play the supportive role in your running, and you will see that as time progress, and as your muscle system becomes stronger, you will have fewer injuries, and your speed and endurance will increase.

I usually do 2 to 3 times alternative exercises and weightlifting in one session or mixed. I follow the FIRST training program for the alternative activities which is either swimming, rowing, or cycling either static or outside. Now I don't know how to swim and even if I knew, I would make no use of it as I live in the mountains, so no time for me to go to a swimming pool or the sea just to train. However, I use the rowing machine, do some cycling at home, and ride my mountain bike whenever I have adequate time apart from the weightlifting.

Tip number 9: Have at least one rest day a week.

I say 'at least' because sometimes when the mileage is accumulating, and the kilograms on the strengthening exercises are adding up, you will see on your own that you need to rest two days, sometimes even three. OH, I know I just "sinned" by saying that, but yes, sometimes you need to take a step back from running to rest, heal, repair, and rejuvenate your storage both physically and mentally.

Now, what are you going to do on your rest days is up to you. I do just that; I rest; I do something entirely different from running or weightlifting. I don't even do yoga; I just relax and unwind. I am a lazy person once a week, and judge me all you want, but it works for me; next day, I feel recharged physically, and, most importantly, my spirit is lifted, and I feel just plain fantastic.

For other people, their version of a rest day is not to run 21km, but 10km! Or they go for cycling or do another alternative exercise like swimming or rowing. Some do Yoga or stretching exercises; other do 30 minutes of weightlifting instead of 1 hour.

Every person is unique, as I said so many times in my books, also in my articles here, my YouTube channel and in other hosting blogs.

The important element to get from this tip is that whatever your rest day contains, the necessary is to get some meaningful rest both physical and emotional; you must get out of the rest day feeling positive   about   yourself.

Tip number 10: Incorporate Hill Training at least once a week.

Oh yeah, baby! Hill training! I know a lot of you are grabbing their quads right now from the pain. Well, say all you want about hill repeats, but they do deliver strong legs, and since I started doing them, I got fewer injuries, people! I swear to you they work; they make our legs stronger, and we are using our body weight to achieve that, also resulting in stronger bones as long you eat enough calcium in your diet to cover your daily needs, you get stronger bones and more muscular glutes and quads; the workforce muscles in running.

What I usually do is start with one hill repeat of 500 meters the first week of my training and keep adding one repeat with each week. When I reach 12 repeats, then I start adding weight on my vest. I have a special vest that you can add 250 grams of sandbags. Four weeks before the race, I start doing fewer hill repeats by removing three repeats every week, so in the last week, I do not do any repeats because I am usually carb loading by then.

I do about 2 miles of the easy run as a proper warm up; then I do the hill repeats, and then I do 2 miles easy as a cool down period again.

Tip number 11: Design a flexible training plan.

When I first started running, I didn't have a training plan because my goal was not to participate in races or achieve any personal records; my goal was a single-minded one, and it was to lose weight, I wanted to lose many kilos and then, in all honesty, I was going to stop running.

I saw running as a way of getting back to my healthy weight, as a mean to an end, and not as something long-term or even a lifestyle.

Well, I lost enough kilos, about 20 of them, but while doing that, I fell in love with running again; I was a runner of 1000 meters, 1500 meters, and 6 km in high school, so I started entering to compete in races.

Now let me tell you why you need to have a flexible training plan. When I registered for my first half-marathon, I just went and ran it! I didn't have a training plan for it; I was running long runs almost every day, that was my training! 2010 races were all like that. I would just run long runs every day and enter in half-marathon races.

In 2011, after seeking to improve my personal record, I started looking into training plans and other types of exercises.

So, after looking around for a while, I downloaded a training schedule, a generic one, from a site on how to train for half-marathon, and I followed that plan to the letter.

I did finish the race faster than the previous times, so I assumed this training program was for me. What I didn't calculate and take into consideration was the fact that I had many injuries during my training. Also, I missed a lot of running days, and lastly, I was feeling like having to go to work when I was following that program.

Anyway, another year went by, and 2012 came, and I decided that reading only online info about training programs would not help me anymore, so I went online and bought a lot of books about running.

I know that, for my regular readers, what I am going to say is a cliché, but every human being on this planet is unique, with different goals and way of thinking, with incomparable life. Some have families; others are alone, and so on. So, a training program, in a nutshell, should serve you and not the other way around, you should create a training program that would improve your life and not hinder it; that will deliver health and happiness and not injuries and bad karma. A training program that will not mess up with your work, family life, friends, and relatives; that will flow along with your inner thoughts and mindset.

Now, how do you achieve that? Well, it is called 'setting priorities.' I must say that, for the brief time I was married, a challenge had risen for me on when I should train. Being alone, having no one to depend on you or worry about, is much easier. Having a g/f, wife and of course kids is much harder to prepare a training plan that will keep the balances of your life together, it's possible, though; I know a lot of moms that run ultra-marathons pushing their kids with them in a baby carriage.

Every year here in Cyprus, on many races, I regularly see a dad running and driving his twin kids along the way, and he always kicks my ass as he finishes faster than me!

I can't tell you how to make the program, but I can tell you what I do and maybe you get some tips or think something that you never thought trying before.

If I am training for a marathon or 50km, I do my running after seven p.m., when I have finished with work and house chores. It might not simulate exactly the race day conditions, but at least I am getting the mileage in, and that's what is important.

On Saturday or Sunday, I do my long runs, and I usually do it in the morning if nothing unexpected occurs.

I do not run every day, I run one day, do strengthening, or weightlifting exercises the next day, and run the other day again. This way, I can switch between exercise regimes. For example, let's say I didn't manage to go for my tempo run on Monday, but I have time to weight lift for 30 minutes. I will do that and next day I will do the tempo run.

I do plan for all the weeks of the training session until race day, but now, what I do is every Sunday about an hour before I go to bed, I sit down and write on the next week's training plan, possible mishaps that might happen, and how to deal with it. This gives me an extra security and a backup plan that I will be ok with my running, and I won't fell off my target goals for the race.

Tip number 12: Make small changes to your training.

If you are running more than a year, you probably are familiar with expressions and phrases like, track repeats, tempo run; long run, threshold runs; VO2 max runs, hill training; fartlek and so many other beautiful exercises and techniques so many runners around the world employ and apply in their everyday training.

Usually, a typical training plan that involves from 5km to a marathon has three main different runs. You have your track repeats, which help you develop your speed; tempo runs, which enable you to build your threshold limit; and lastly, long runs, which make your body conditioned for endurance. So, we have speed, pace, and endurance, three elements a runner must develop to have the best success.

There is also hill training and fartlek, *fartlek* is a Swedish word, and it means 'speed play.' You run with a certain speed, usually during your tempo runs, and you decide for a period or a certain distance to go faster and keep that pace. After that, you return to your initial pace, and you do this without any programmed way.

What this training achieves is to build endurance when someone is trying to overpower you, you are conditioning your body to hold your position and beat him/her if needed. It makes your body adaptive to different speeds during the race.

Hill repeats or hill training is another exercise all runners should incorporate at some point in their regime. Hills make our legs stronger, thus reducing the possibility of injuries.

One week you might have the three primary runs and some hill training, and the next week same three again, plus some fartlek exercises.

The important thing here to remember is to listen to your body and make small changes every week. I will give you a few examples, so you get what I mean by this.

Let's say you just finished a long run, a 13-mile run (21 km), that's a half-marathon distance, and you were out of breath the last few kilometers, you really struggled to finish.

Next week you have an even bigger long run, what would you do? Would you follow the program, or would you listen to your body?

Another example: you were doing track repeats, and you noticed that even that you are trying to maintain a certain pace for your loops, you seem to finish them faster than what you originally planned, and when done, you felt that you can make some more. What would you do? Would you increase your speed the following week or stick to the program that says to keep the same speed?

Of course, you would listen to your body. The following week, you would not increase the long run's distance, you maintain the same or even reduce it; nothing shameful about that.

Also, next week, you would go at a faster pace because your body is telling you to do so.

The secret is trying to do one change per week, and always try to make either a distance change or a speed change. Do not make two changes either distance or speed in a week, or it will mess up with your body's recovery and adaptation times.

MAKE only one change every week. Give your body able time to adapt and recover and always −always − listen to your body. Never allow yourself to become a slave of a training program and follow it to the letter. We are human beings with life that changes every day, not robots in an assembly machine that must keep a schedule.

Tip number 13: Train with friends.

This advice – let's just call it a suggestion – is a double edge blade. I tried both ways, running alone and with company. Training alone has more chances of success if you have self-discipline, and you are consistent.

Training with a friend is highly dependent on whether both of you have the same level of fitness, are training for the same distance or race, and both of you have and share similar and precise goals of why you are running. If one of the above situations is slightly different, problems will arise down the road.

If one of you is training for a 5km and the other for a half-marathon, then there will be inconsistencies and disagreement on the distance and the time you will train. Therefore, it won't be easy to train together.

So, if you are going to train with a friend, make sure you share the same general running goals. Otherwise, it is better to train alone.

On the other hand, if both of you, or more of you, train for the same race and have the same level of fitness, then the support you will get from each other, and the lessons you will learn from each other are invaluable. It is an amazing feeling the comradeship that is developed as it happens with every awesome start of many everlasting friendships between people.

Tip number 14: Participate as often as you can in races.

My advice when you are starting to get bored in your everyday running is that it's time to improve your game and consider participating in races.

It will open a whole new way of viewing running, and it will expand your horizons. For starters, you will find out that you are not alone in this world. Participating in an official race, where you will get your finisher's medal, you are officially a runner. You just joined the craziest, bizarre, and beautiful tribe of the entire world, ***the runner's tribe***!

You can consider yourself a runner from now on; not an amateur runner or a recreational runner or, even worse, a "Jogger."

You can only gain positive results and benefits by running in an official race. Just by observing other athletes of all levels, from the fat lady that wants to lose weight to the elite runner that wants to come first place and make a record; from the beginner to the moms and dads running with their kids, you can learn something from each one of them that you can use and benefit from.

You can see how they warm up; what kind of exercises they use; how much time they spend warming up and when they start their warmup; when they use the toilet and when they go to position themselves on the starting line; what kind of shoes they wear, clothes, hats; what kind of sunblock they use and what kind of glasses they wear.

Are they carrying water with them? Electrolytes or both, are they using watches to track their progress, GPS watches, and pacemakers? There are so many other little devices that make up a runner that you will only see if you participate in a race and observe.

Personally, I learned a lot from taking part in sports. I found out that you stitch your number on the front of your t-shirt and not on the back like I did on my first back in 2010. I also learned the importance of a good warmup period before running.

Learned how to refuel properly from the aid stations that are situated in strategical spots along the route of the race.

I made a ton of friends while running in races, strong friendships with people from all the countries I went and ran.

Do not deny yourself the opportunity to experience what it means to be part of a running race.

Now every weekend, there are races all around the globe. I am sure if you search, you can even find one that is very close to where you live. Find more, participate, make a running plan, follow it, and finish that race.

Tip number 15: Read a lot of books about running.

When I decided that I wanted to do something more than just running around my high school track like a hamster, I realized that I didn't know anything about how to train properly and how to condition my body to be ready for an official event as a race. Also, I had no idea what to eat during training periods. Should I eat differently? Should I eat more, less? I was completely at lost.

So, one of the first things I did was to go online and go to my favorite place where I buy books namely Amazon and get a lot of books about running!

I can say that all of them helped me a lot, and some of them are still until today providing valuable information on anything I want to know on how, when, where and what to eat and train.

I stopped using ready training plans that I found on the internet, and with the help of these books and with my progressive experience, I started making my customized running training schedules and plans.

Don't get me wrong; I am glad that I used those ready ones that I found online; they helped me at the beginning when I didn't know anything about athletic performance and athletic nutrition, I am still learning about these subjects, I just know a bit more than I used to, and that's the beauty of running; the flexibility that it offers will keep my curiosity and my motivation engaged for years to come.

Now and then, new things are popping up, new ways to train, new ways to eat, new exercises, and methods that provide better results, and so on. It's a constant fluctuation as running is concerned, and I love it.

The following list of books I highly recommend if you are serious about your running.

Books that I highly recommend!

1.   CHI RUNNING by Danny Dreyer and Katherine Dreyer

2.   COMPLETE BOOK ABOUT RUNNING edited by Amby Burfoot

3.   BEYOND THE IRON by Wayne Kurtz

4.   EAT & RUN by Scott Jurek with Steve Friedman

5.   FINDING ULTRA by Rich Roll

6.   GALLOWAY'S BOOK ON RUNNING 2nd edition by Jeff Galloway.

7.   GOING LONG edited by David Willey

8.   HOW TO TRAIN AND FINISH YOUR FIRST 5K RACE by Andreas Michaelides

9.   HOW RUNNING SAVED MY LIFE by Andreas Michaelides

10.   ONCE A RUNNER by John L. Parker, Jr

11.   POSE METHOD OF RUNNING by Nicholas Romanov, Ph.D.

12.   RUNNING & PHILOSOPHY edited by Michael W. Austin

13.   RUN THE MIND-BODY METHOD OF RUNNING BY FEEL BY Matt Fitzgerald

14.   THE RUNNER'S BODY by Ross Tucker, Ph.D. and Jonathan Dugas , Ph.D. with Matt Fitzgerald

15.   RUNNING THE LYDIARD WAY by Arthur Lydiard with Garth Gilmour

16.   RUNNING THE SACRED ART Dr. Warren A. Kay

17.   RUNNING THROUGH THE WALL BY Neal Jamison

18.   RUNNING WITH THE BUFFALOES by Chris Lear

19.   RUN LESS RUN FASTER by Bill Pierce. Scott Murr and Ray Moss

20.   RUNNING ANATOMY by Joe Puleo and Dr. Patrick Milroy

21.   SPARTAN UP by Joe De Sena

22.   THE RUNNER'S YOGA BOOK by Jean Couch

23.   THE COMPETITIVE RUNNER'S HANDBOOK by Bob Glover and Shelly-lynn Florence Glover

24.   THE NON-RUNNER'S MARATHON TRAINER by David A. Whitsett, Forrest A. Dolgener ann Tanjala Mabon Kole

25.   THE RUNNER'S RULE BOOK by Mark Remy

26.   THRIVE FITNESS by Brendan Brazier

27.   WHAT I TALK ABOUT WHEN I TALK ABOUT RUNNING by Haruki Murakami

Tip number 16: Create a running Blog/log to track your progress.

When I started running again in 2010, one of the first things I started keeping was a running log where I would input how many meters I walked and ran.

I kept that running log for three years, and it was one of the best things I've ever done in my life. By keeping track of your running progress, you create a dynamic tool that will help you extremely in the future.

It may not seem much keeping a diary, it may even sound girly, but I assure you, there is nothing girly about that.

A running diary or a log will make you remember why you started running in the first place. When you feel sad or overwhelmed, you can always open that log and check what your situation was in the past, and you will see an immediate rejuvenation in you because you will understand what you have accomplished all this time, and it will give you the strength and the willpower not to give up on running.

Also, another aspect that a log can help you with is tracking your performance and finding out which exercise works best for you, how many repetitions of a particular training is better for you, etc.

When and in which order you should do another kind of training are questions that a diary will be capable of answering, and you can use it as your base to make better adjustments in the future to increase your performance even more.

A diary's like having a friend checking your running from a distance and letting you know what you did wrong or right or what you need to fix or work on.

Also, my running log helped me remember episodes in my life that I later used in my first book *Thirsty for Health* when I was writing the chapter about running.

You can make even a more daring step, something that I never had the will or the courage to do, but you can totally do it if you like the idea. You can make an online running blog where you can catalog there and post about how your training is going.

This way you add to your weaponry the asset of not failing in front of all those people that will read your blog. It's an added motivation to keep going, bettering yourself so you won't let down not only yourself but also your readers and followers; a way to keep yourself accountable.

Plus, by having an online blog, you can have a greater opportunity of interacting and making friends with other running bloggers, thus increasing your chances of acquiring valuable information from fellow running bloggers about anything you can think of, like training tactics, nutrition plans, gears, and shoes you can use the sky is the limit.

WordPress is a very easy and free way to set up a blog without too much trouble and with not much computer knowledge.

Tip number 17: Create a food log to track your progress.

As I said before, the only reason I started running again back in 2010 was to lose weight, and as soon as I would shake the extra weight off, I would stop. Somewhere along the way, though, I fell in love with running again and stuck with it, and I am glad I did!

Now, back then, I didn't track my calories intake, and that was one of the reasons that for at least two years my weight stayed unchanged.

In 2013, though, when I decided to make the transition from an omnivore to a 100% plant-based diet and later the lifestyle, I started keeping a food log because I had to supplement the calories I was taking as an omnivore from animal-based food with plant-based.

It was one of the best things that I did because the food diary, pretty much like the running log described earlier, gave me information that I could use to better my nutrition both in quantity and quality, which would allow me to support a vigorous training regime like training for a marathon.

I found out which foods were causing gas or heartburn, or they would upset my stomach. I knew what quantities to have a particular food. I improved the food combinations I was making and so many other aspects, like detecting which food helped me with defecation or gave me diarrhea or constipation, which food to eat before a training session, which to eat after, and so on.

Having a food diary motivates you to learn more information about nutrition and how this impacts your running and your health in general.

What I concluded, health wise speaking is that 85% is nutrition and 15% is exercise. That's how important nutrition is for our health and our quality of life.

You can keep it handwritten or computerized on a word processor, or you can use online food logs like www.cromoner.com which is the one I use as well.

A small search online will provide you with a plethora of similar food catalog engines. It's up to you to find the one that is to your liking and adopt it.

Tip number 18: Learn more about nutrition and especially running nutrition.

I know that sometimes I come across as a broken record, and I apologize in advance if I repeat episodes from my life over and over, but it's important for me to put some items in perspective in order for you to better understand my points and to see with your own eyes that the tips I offer come from my life experience and not from a random search on the internet.

As I said before, back in 2010 when I started running again, running was a way to lose weight, and then I would stop doing it, after losing the pounds, 44 of them! But I fell in love with running all over again – I was an athlete runner back in high school.

When I reached a plateau in my personal records, I did not give up. I started researching other aspects that could help me improve and optimize my running personal records, and I did what I knew best; I went online and bought a lot of books about nutrition and running. Some of them were excellent, and I still consult them daily while others were not so great.

So, I found out that if I were going to adopt a plant-based diet, I would have the chance to improve my running times, and so I did. The first year was a disaster; I was always hungry, sleepy, tired; my energy levels were plummeting, and I didn't know what I was doing wrong.

That's when my food diary and my running diary came in handy as they provided the solution to my problem.

My mistake was that I did not replace the calories adequately, the ones I was not getting from animal products with plant-based ones, and second, I increased my exercise level. Roughly, I needed 3000 calories every day, and I was consuming only 2500!

Once I satisfied my calorie intake, all the things I read about the plant-based benefits started to kick in.

I was recovering faster; I didn't have to sleep eight hours; six were enough; I could train more because I could recover faster.

This is my experience with nutrition, I am sure the best thing you can do is experiment with different lifestyles and diets, and you will see what is best for you.

The important thing I want you to know is you should be able always to question everything and anytime. Do not assume that what you learn today is always valid, things change every time, and you should keep up with new knowledge. That's what running is, it's a fluctuated movement that demands open minds and inquiring brains.

Nutrition is 85% and exercises 15% in my book, and that's what I learned thus far from my experimentation and all the books (written by doctors), articles (written by doctor and researchers) and all the video presentations (made by doctors again).

Tip number 19: Start doing Yoga.

I know a lot of people will say Yoga is useless or doesn't offer anything, well, I must admit I was thinking like them a few years ago that yoga was a waste of time, time that I could use to run more. Then again, when I first started running, I thought warming up and cooling down were a waste of time too until I got some semi-serious injuries and learned the hard way. Same thing with weightlifting and strengthening exercises, at some point, I thought they were a waste of time too! Now, I lift three times a week.

The reason I thought all things was a waste of time is that I was swimming in sweet ignorance. I didn't know anything about running. I assumed I knew; that's our biggest mistake. Well like as Everett McGill in the movie with Steven Seagal *"Under Siege 2: Dark Territory* in the train said: '**Assumption is the mother of all fuckups!**'

Do not assume, search and research, apply and experiment, have results, find what works for you and apply it until you accomplish a relative perfection.

I assumed Yoga was a waste of time. After getting a serious injury on my right leg on my ITB, I started doing rehabilitation exercises on my own, from exercises, I found online, and that one thing led to another, and I did what I always do best, I bought a few books about yoga and started educating myself.

It turns out Yoga has a lot of similarities and common aspects with my mindset. Yoga philosophy as Greek Philosophers and my ancestors, in general, did not consider the brain to be the most important aspect of a person; they saw its wholeness of body, mind, and spirit. They didn't try to train only one and leave the others behind; they had gymnasiums where they will go to train; they invented the Olympic Games for goodness's sake; we had the theater and arts. All the ancient Greek statues are full of beauty and show how my ancestors saw the human body; strong, healthy, with muscles everywhere, radiating health and happiness.

Today's society only trains our brain. You know it from our educational system, from elementary to university, we train the mind, educate, learn information; we don't give the proper attention to the other two aspects of our existence; body and spirit. Athletics in schools is not as developed and promoted, and don't let me start about the cultivation of the spirit.

Yoga, like ancient Greek Philosophy, combines all these three important parts of a human being and tries to bring balance to them and, in conclusion, to us.

The slow static exercises of yoga give you the time to connect with your body and discover your muscles in your body.

It helps our body to relax, to develop a better elasticity and flexibility making injuries very rare to occur.

Alignment of the body using the various yoga exercises allows for the body to accommodate better breathing.

Also, the breathing exercises of yoga enable the strengthening of the lungs, thus receiving oxygen faster and more efficient.

You feel more relaxed after a yoga session, more balanced, more in tune with yourself.

My advice is to incorporate it slowly into your life; you don't have to be a runner to benefit from yoga.

I use exercises from the Hatha Yoga which, after a lousy translation, means Yoga for Health, and that is what I aim for always; I am always thirsty for health.

All I can say is that since I started doing about 45 minutes of Yoga once a week, usually either Saturday or Sunday, I feel much better; my back pain is gone, injuries do not bother me as they used to; I feel relaxed and without stress, and I do feel I am in control of my life.

Try it yourself! You have nothing to lose but everything to gain.

Tip number 20: Use swimming as an alternative exercise to running.

One of the many good books I bought about running is Run Less Run Faster by Bill Pierce, Scott Murr, and Ray Moss. This book was a life saver for me because it showed me that I could run less and achieve faster time on my races.

Its philosophy, in a nutshell, is run three times a week and two times a week engage in an alternative exercise. One of those exercises is swimming. Swimming is an excellent complimentary for your running.

Unfortunately for me I see two disadvantages as swimming is concerned. First, I don't know how! And second, I live on the mountain, and the nearest proper swimming pool is 40 minutes away by car.

So, I do not engage in this wonderful exercise, but if you live near the sea or a lake or have the time to visit a swimming pool, then you should incorporate swimming as a cross training exercise that will help improve your running.

Usually, swimming is adopted by runners and other sportsmen when they have an injury that prevents them from indulging themselves in the act of running.

The reason that they choose swimming is that of its low impact on the body and especially on the legs, this way you maintain your fitness level and give time to the injured part of your body to recover from an injury or a hard run like a long run for example.

Swimming increases mostly the upper body; it provides a strong core which is essential in running while at the same time takes much of the stress off the legs giving them the chance to recover and heal faster from previous running training.

In swimming, only 10% of the propulsion comes from the legs which except giving them a much-needed rest as I mentioned it makes them more flexible, the hamstrings and the ankles develop a better elasticity and flexibility, thus improving the running performance and reducing at the same time the risk of leg injuries. The more flexible your body is the least injuries you will suffer.

Like any sports, swimming, especially, demands from you good form and technique to be able to get a good cardio workout.

If you insist on swimming as an alternative exercise regime, you will see that it will be rewarding in the end as your running performance is concerned. Plan and experiment with it.

If you are like me, and you don't know how to swim, ask a friend that knows how to swim or hire a swimming trainer to teach you. In the future, when I will have more time available, I will do that; I will go register for swimming lessons and incorporate it into my running training. As you get older, especially, you will want to maintain the same fitness level with the least impact on your body, and especially on your legs.

Aim to exercise swimming for 30 minutes and set to achieve goals that cover certain distances. For example, aim to swim non-stop for 400 meters and start increasing them until 1500 meters.

Tip number 21: Use Cycling as an alternative exercise to running.

Contrary to the fact that I don't know how to swim, I think even before I started walking, I was cycling. I remember my siblings and me doing endless rounds with our bikes around the house driving our parents nuts many times because we would not stop even for food, that's how much fun we were having with our bikes.

The same reasoning as swimming applies for cycling too. It's an amazing alternative to running training.

It's a no-weight bearing and low impact sport on the legs. It develops aerobic capacity and fitness while at the same time gives the opportunity to the legs to rest, heal and recover.

Cycling's low impact can be observed on cyclists that have been training since their teens and now have obvious symptoms of osteopenia which means weak, brittle bones. That's why it's important, if you only cycle as a sport, to do weightlifting as well because weightlifting makes our bones stronger.

Cycling except for offering the aerobic fitness and the low leg impact, it strengthens the quadriceps bringing balance on the legs because of running's ability to develop the hamstrings and the calves more than the quadriceps. So, with running, you are developing the quadriceps bringing balance to the whole leg.

While swimming develops the flexibility of the lower leg and the ankles, cycling develops hip and knee joint flexibility which is important in running.

Doing interval cycling improves the leg turnover for running, making us faster. High power bike intervals work the leg muscles harder and more intense than doing hill repeats without the brutal impact hill running applies to the legs.

For the runner that use the bike to improve their performance is a good tactic to maintain 80 to 90 rpm (revolutions per minute) for strength workouts and 90 to 100 rpm for tempo and recovery sessions.

What kind of cycling you will do depends on a lot of issues. If you are an extrovert and more social person, then outdoor cycling is better for you.

Outdoor cycling has some disadvantages, though. It costs more than running as equipment is concerned (buy a good bike, helmet, uniform, flashlight, etc.) Also, you need to take into consideration the traffic and the fact that there are many stupid drivers out there. Also, weather condition could be brutal and increase the possibility of having an accident that could injure you severely. Especially bad weather conditions like raining, windy, and snowing increase the danger of having an accident. Also, when you cycle outside, you may have a flat tire, and you will lose time to change it.

Now, indoor cycling on a stationary bike has more advantages than disadvantages. First, is safer, second, it could be social and fun if you are exercising in a gym. Furthermore, the weather is not an issue for you, so you don't have to worry about that. Also, you don't have to worry about reckless automobile drivers.

Plus, while you cycle indoors, you can listen to music, watch a movie, or even read a book.

Personally, I use both, but I mostly use the indoor bike to train. I rarely use my mountain bike because I want to utilize as much time as I can, and since 2012, when I had a severe mountain bike accident, I only use the mountain bike whenever I miss having a race in the forest.

Tip number 22: Use Rowing as an alternative exercise to running.

Like swimming, I never had the opportunity to row in the sea or a facility that enables rowing, but unlike swimming, there are a lot of various rowing machines you can use if you are a member of a gym or buy one like I did, and you don't fancy going to the gym. I prefer to exercise at home to my private gym I have set up myself. I bought a traditional rowing machine with the handles, and I am very pleased with it.

Rowing is a total body non-weight bearing exercise, and it works both the lower and upper body. In my book, it's the perfect exercise because it combines the legs that you train more with cycling and the core that you can train with swimming! So, I try to use my rowing machine as often as I can in my training plans.

It's a total body workout exercise for all our muscles, goes through various and different motions, and this promotes total body flexibility, thus reducing possible future injuries while running.

Because its indoors, it can be done anywhere and anytime. I try to incorporate 30 minutes of rowing a week in my plan, and it's amazing because it's self-paced, meaning you decide how fast or slow you will train.

Tip number 23: Build your aerobic capacity first.

One of the first books I read about running and about training was "Running the Lydiard Way" by Arthur Lydiard with Garth Gilmour.

The author advocated that before you start doing any strengthening exercise, it's important to build your aerobic capacity first and when you bring it to the desired level, then start doing threshold training, CO_2 training, etc.

Of course, the book was written years ago and a zillion new techniques and methods of training in running were developed and are still developing, but I, personally, like this notion of first building the aerobic state and until today, when I have the time, I apply this principle that was first used by Arthur Lydiard so many years ago.

You run at a comfortable pace, around 60 to 70% of your maximum heart rate, and you increase the mileage slowly until you reach the aerobic level you desire and is mainly based on the distance you are training for.

Lydiard was famous for training his 800-meter athletes with 90 minutes long aerobic runs and 10km time trial exercises!

I always train to build my aerobic limit, which is the limit where I can breathe in, transport, and use oxygen with ease. After that point, the anaerobic metabolism kicks in, and oxygen is not the only fuel that is used to produce energy from the muscles.

My advice and from my experience are to build your aerobic state first and then start incorporating the other different training exercises.

Tip number 24: Build a strong upper body (core).

When I first started running again back in 2010, I foolishly believed that I knew everything I needed to know about running; the sad truth was that I didn't know anything. The result of my ignorance was repeated injuries that left me out of running for several months.

I was under the impression that warming up and cooling down was a waste of time I also thought that rest days were a waste of good running too. That had their toll on me. The last ignorant castle that fell in my mind was that the upper body doesn't play any role in running. I was under the false impression that you only need a good pair of strong legs for running. I was wrong, of course, again.

After the injuries, I made it my goal to build a strong upper body, to develop a fit core able to carry me through all the 26 miles of a marathon.

A strong upper core provides balance and stability to our running, supports, and supplements it, and increases our lung capacity by enlarging our rib cage.

Now, I train three times a week by lifting weights and doing other strengthening exercises. I am not going to have any more injuries anymore because of stupidity, ignorance, and lack of self-knowledge.

Tip number 25: Define why are you running.

It is vital to know before you start running or start training, why you are going to do it. I mean, you must have a clear target, a precise goal of why. This way you'll be able to design a plan which if you follow, it will bring the best optimization of your efforts.

For example, back in 2010, when I started running to lose weight, I didn't have any other goal in mind, I wasn't interested in participating in any races at that moment in my life. So, I had a clear-cut goal for what I wanted, and that was to lose weight.

If you want to start running to lose weight, then a slow pace running near to your 60% of your maximum heart rate is ideal because it's the pace where you are in your aerobic state, and it's the state that you burn fat as a fuel than glucose.

If you are interested in running so you can participate in races, then you must exercise at least three kinds of runs, track repeats to build speed, tempo runs to build threshold endurance, and long runs to build endurance and aerobic strength.

Knowing in advance what do you want out of running will make it a happy experience for you. It will not be stressful because you know exactly what you want. It's ok to experiment at the beginning to realize what you want from running, but something I learned the hard way is that you shouldn't try to achieve two goals at the same time.

At some point, I was trying to lose weight and improve my personal athletic records. However, it didn't go quite as I expected. The two goals were clashing with each other; I didn't lose more weight, and I didn't improve my PR. So, be clear about what you want out of running, and you'll be on the right track of having an activity that you will never get bored, always enjoy, learn more and more through this and, at the end, build up your self-confidence and self-esteem because you will achieve your goals.

Tip number 26: Do regular health checkups.

This is one of the most important things you should do at least once a year. Checking your blood, cholesterol, blood pressure, thyroid, your minerals like iron, electrolytes like sodium, is a must. It will give you a good picture of how healthy you are internally, and it will also show you how much running has improved your health. Then, you will not have any more excuses but continue running and adopt running or any other kind of exercise as a lifestyle.

As I mentioned many times six years ago, my intention was to stop running after I lost the extra weight, but, in the meantime, I fell in love with running again, and I continue it. Except for falling in love with it, my new blood results were also so much better than the last years when I was still a lazy person. So, seeing firsthand what a tremendous healthy benefit the running had on my body was another motivation for me not to stop running.

With that been said, you too should make a checkup at least once a year; except your health, you can get an enormous psychological boost from the improvements you will see with your own eyes in black and white on your lab results papers.

Tip number 27: Make friends with other runners.

I am an introvert at heart, and even that I worked hard not to show it and still do, in my everyday social interactions, there is still this kid in me shouting, "get a book and let's go into our room and read and leave all these people."

Running helped me make some wonderful friends and acquaintances. Making friends with other runners, you open yourself to a huge bank of information that it would take you years to accumulate through reading books or articles or from personal experimentation.

Spending 30 minutes with other runners, you can pick up knowledge that, as I said, would, otherwise, take you considerable time to find out. We, runners, are a very sharing tribe. If something worked for us, such as a specific exercise or nutrition or anything else that has helped our running – either mental or a pair of shoes – we will pass on that information and share it with the other fellow runners. Because let's face it, they are the only ones that will appreciate and cherish the information.

So here you have it; making friends with other runners helps you learn a lot of information about running in a very short period.

Second, having runners as friends can help you with your training. Also, if they live near you, they can inform you about new races or other race events.

They can be there for you when your life is not that great. They can help you better because they know what it means to wake up at four in the morning to run a few miles before the spouse, and the kids wake up or wait until everybody goes to sleep before going for a few laps around the block or around a track nearby.

Making running buddies will ensure that you go the long distance without giving up running until it becomes a lifestyle for you. Then, at some point, when through experimentation and experience you can transmit knowledge to a newbie runner, you will have completed the cycle!

Tip number 28: Keep a detailed activity log of your races.

Some of you might not see the usefulness of this tip. Well, let me try to change your mind. I think that there will be a time in the future where you will want to enter and compete again in the same race as a few years go or even a few months ago, and you will want to do better this time.

Unfortunately, you will not remember exactly how you trained the previous time, what food you ate, what exercises you did, and most of all, you won't remember your time records.

By keeping a detailed activity log while you are training for a race and saving it, it will help you in the future to achieve better personal records because you will have a base which you can build on. You will not have to start designing the plan from scratch again, and, by correcting mistakes and errors you made you will improve other aspects of your training, you'll be able to achieve a better running time next time.

It's smart to keep an activity log; in the future, if you want to write a book, then you can use that log to remember and get advice from it. That's what I did with my first book; for the running chapter, I used my race activity logs to get information, that I incorporated in the book.

All I can say is better to have one than none. It's your call at the end.

Tip number 29: Do one track session a week.

It doesn't matter if you are training for a 5km or a 50km, you need to train to optimize your speed, especially for races from 5km to half-marathon. You need to improve your maximum VO_2 running speed and running economy. Now, what is a maximum VO_2, you might ask, and you'll be right asking it. In very simple terms, VO_2 is the ability of an athlete to produce energy using oxygen as a fuel; this is called aerobic system, status, method, and so on. If your muscles produce energy (ATP) using glucose and oxygen, then you are in the aerobic state, and it's good because it's this state that your body- except glucose - can use fat as fuel to propel you forward. You need to increase this limit as much as possible because when you reach that limit, then the second system kicks in which is called anaerobic, and in this system, muscles start to use lactate instead of oxygen to produce energy (ATP).

Track sessions or otherwise known interval training achieves to increase your max VO_2 limit which will have as a result for you to be able to perform more work.

The intensity of your track repeats should be the same as your 5km race pace or a little bit faster than that and the duration should be 10 minutes or less.

Running Economy is also improved with training intervals because you learn how to use your body and practice on the right form of running. There is an excellent book called *The Running Pose* written by Nicholas Romanov, Ph.D. that shows what kind of exercises you can do to achieve running economy.

Tip number 30: Do one Tempo session a week.

Now, tempo runs do play a different role; they improve your endurance dramatically by raising lactate threshold.

Lactate is a by-product of anaerobic metabolism, by doing tempo runs, you train yourself not to reach your LT by running at 50 to 60% of your heart rate.

By doing tempo runs, your muscles are trained to do endurance like work. Also, the accumulation of lactate in the blood is an indicator of how intensely a runner can go for certain periods of time, usually 30 minutes or more.

Your tempo should be hard, but at the same time comfortable. They should be 15 to 45 seconds slower from your 5km pace race, and it should be about 20 to 45 minutes long at certain rhythm and tempo pace.

Tip number 31: Do your long run during the weekend.

Depending on the day where the race will be held, Saturday or Sunday, try to do your long run the day of the race to accustom your body to run on that specific day and acclimatize it, train it to run that day of the week.

With long runs, we improve endurance by raising aerobic metabolism, meaning, we can run more time using oxygen to burn glucose or fat to produce energy that will catapult us forward.

The intensity of the run should be about 30 seconds slower than your marathon pace goal, and it should be about an hour to three hours long.

Tip number 32: Watch Documentaries about running.

There are dozens of documentaries out there about running. I always try to watch them when I have some free time because watching the success or the failures of fellow runners helps me to learn a lot.

Also, it is a tremendous source of inspiration, watching a documentary about a man that ran 50 marathons in 50 states in 50 days or a small Indian boy who run 48 marathons by the age of four!!! Documentaries bring to my attention and into my life unbelievable stories but at the same time humane tales of incredible endurance.

Documentaries will give you the opportunity to learn a lot about running, even at a subconscious level, which is always wonderful when it happens. One day you are doing a new personal record, or you are perfecting a specific training exercise, and you are wondering how did I just did that? Well, it's your subconscious feeding you with knowledge when it feels that you are ready to receive it and utilize it to the optimum level.

Here are ten documentaries in alphabetical order that you should watch.

1. Marathon Boy

2. Personal Best

3. Run For Your Life

4. Running on the Sun: The Badwater 135

5. Running The Sahara

6. Spirit of the Marathon

7. Steve Prefontaine: Fire on the Track

8. Town of Runners

9. The Dipsea Demon

10. Ultramarathon Man

Tip number 33: Watch Movies about running.

Same principal as the previous tip with the bonus that you can have a little bit more fun and entertainment along the side. I love movies that are biographical, that they illustrate the life of a runner, like Steve Prefontaine.

There is something magical about movies, especially when a film is about a running event like the Olympic Games. *Chariots of Fire* – what an amazing movie – if you want to name yourself a runner, you should watch the film.

Movies will inspire you to become the best runner you can be. Music and theatrics combined will lift your soul to new heights of knowledge and existence.

If you want to call yourself a runner again, you should watch the following twelve movies listed here in alphabetical order:

1. Chariots of Fire

2. Forrest Gump

3. On the Edge

4. Personal Best

5. Running Brave

6. Run For Your Life

7. Run Lola Run

8. Saint Ralph

9. Spirit of the Marathon

10. The Jericho Mile

11. The Long Green Line

12. Without Limits

Tip number 34: Read inspiring stories about running.

Human beings learn through certain modalities. My modality is visual; I learn more and better if I see something done, or someone is showing me how to do something. Other people are auditory, meaning they learn quicker and better by hearing. Others learn by being tactile, through touch, and last, but not least, there are people who prefer kinesthetic, participating in learning.

All four of these ways are used by us, some to a greater degree, and others to a lesser degree. Reading employs three of the modalities, visual, tactile (you have a book in your hand), and kinesthetic because you are participating in the story you are reading.

By reading books about running, you increase your possibilities of learning three times more, and you can read a book anywhere you are on the bus, on the plane, waiting in line to get your coffee, in the toilet.

Plus, with eBooks now, you can have zillion books on your phone, tablet, or portable computer, and you can read whenever you find some free time.

I especially like stories that have a good ending of course, but I also love stories of people that had a similar background and path towards running as me.

I personally recommend reading the following books, they inspired me, and they still do as running is concerned. I learned so much about running through people telling their stories than books that are more professional and running dedicated.

1.   FINDING ULTRA by Rich Roll

2.   GOING LONG edited by David Willey

3.   HOW RUNNING SAVED MY LIFE by Andreas Michaelides

4.   <u>RUNNING WITH THE BUFFALOES</u> by Chris Lear

5.   <u>WHAT I TALK ABOUT WHEN I TALK ABOUT RUNNING</u> by Haruki Murakami

6.   <u>SIX AWESOME PERSONAL SHORT RUNNING STORIES BY SIX EVERYDAY PEOPLE</u> by <u>Andreas Michaelides</u>

<u>Tip number 35: Learn to be flexible.</u>

If you read one of my previous books about running, either *'<u>How Running saved my life</u>'* or *'<u>How to train and finish your first 5k race</u>'* you will see that when I first started running, I went online and adopted various fixed and ready to go training programs for the distances I wanted to race for, and I followed them to the letter.

Some of them were good, some of them were just plain bad while others were somewhere in the middle.

I did learn a lot from these online programs, and one of them was that I learned to be flexible in a hard way. After a series of serious and minor injuries, I realized that I needed to oversee my program and not to be the slave of the program's commands and demands.

Let me give you an example. As I already mentioned here, one of the tips is to have at least one rest day. I usually have mine on Friday because all the tiredness of the week is really on my shoulders, so the last thing I want to do is either go running or lift weights or do yoga. I just want to sit on my couch, watch a movie having a beer and a big ball of popcorns or read a good book and enjoy a nice red glass of wine.

This doesn't work all the time, though. For example, this week I did my weightlifting on Monday, I did bike and triceps exercises. On Tuesday, I was supposed to do track repeats, but something happened, and I couldn't do them, so instead of hitting myself about it and stressing out that I missed a scheduled training session, I decided that

I will have my rest day on Tuesday, and I'd do something else on Friday.

Another example, on Wednesday, I had scheduled to do weightlifting, but because I lost the Tuesday's session, I did the training session of Tuesday on Wednesday, and I would adjust accordingly as the week progresses.

Also, on Wednesday, I wanted to do the track repeats I missed on Tuesday from 5 p.m. to 6 p.m., but my father came and wanted help with the house, so I went and helped him and did my track repeats after, from 7 a.m. to 8 a.m.

See, you must be ready to allow yourself not to stress about missing training sessions and educate yourself and train and always try to see solutions instead of dead ends, and you'll be fine. Rome was not built in a day, and with practice, you will see you will develop a flexible attitude, not just about running but about your life in general, and that's a good thing. By being flexible, you can face and deal with unexpected situations and come on top of them and all of these because you learned how to be flexible with your running training plan!

If you want to be successful with running, and I don't mean with personal records or finishing or not finishing races, but by adopting running as a lifestyle, you need to be flexible and be able to balance your work, your family, and you're running like an acrobat on a rope without a safety net underneath!

Tip number 36: Have a backup plan.

What I mean by that? Well, I am referring to two things. First, in case your race gets canceled and in case you can't go out to train for your running.

I always plan my races at least 4 months before, and for the place that the race is going to be held, I do detailed research, and I always try to find sightseeing worth visiting if I have time before and after the race. If the race gets canceled or if at the last minute something happens to me and I can't participate, I will always have something to do; go visit a museum, dine in a good restaurant, go out to a nice night club, and so on. Have a backup plan so you won't get disappointed just in case the unthinkable happens.

The other thing is that sometimes you are so tired that you can't go out to do your long run, or it's raining or-or-or, what I do is I am replacing the long run with my static bike. If for example, I must do 16km long run, I do 32km of static cycling instead. This way I achieve two things; I rest my legs by not having them pounding for 16km and at the same time, I keep myself in shape aerobically, and my leg muscles get their share of training.

Also, I can watch a movie while cycling or read a book or listen to nice music.

I am sure there are other events or situations that you can think of, and you should always try to have valid and useful backup plans and backup procedures and functions in place just in case!

Tip number 37: Have a ritual before the day of the race.

No, I am not asking you to do Voodoo or anything, but it's a good thing to build a routine the day before the race. I personally, knowing exactly what I am going to do the day before the race, it calms me down. As a result, my stress is going down, and that allows me to have a good, nice sleep the night before the race so in the next morning, the morning of the race, I'll be fine and rested. I won't be a mental wreck worrying if I packed this or did that and generally stressing about the race.

I always eat at specific times during the day. I eat the same food, food that I tested all these years, and I am sure they will not give me an upset stomach or bloating or anything unpleasant, both the day before and on race day. Looking for a toilet while you are running is not a fun thing to have.

I pack specific stuff. I always have a list of things I take with me. I have it in many copies, so I just pick one copy of my list and tick which items I already packed and which I will pack the day of the race.

I go to bed at a specific time, and I always have my herbal tea 30 minutes before I go to bed.

Your routine might be like mine, but I am sure it will have its differences, and that's completely natural. As I said a lot of time in my books and on my articles on my blog, we are unique and of course, your pre-race day will be unique also, and it will be yours!

Tip number 38: Have a ritual the day of the race.

Like the previous tip, having a ritual on race day will help you calm down, it will give you something to do, all that stress will be channeled through your ritual, having as a result again to reduce your stress about the race.

I always wake up 3 hours before the race. I make sure all the stuff I need for the race are in my running bag. I make sure I use the toilet several times to know I am empty, so I won't be having any accidents while running.

I will go to the race place at least an hour before the race starts. I will make sure I change, use the toilet, do my warm-up, and go get a good starting position at the race start.

Don't worry; after participating in a few races, you will see what works best for you and adopt it and what is not working for you, you will either reject it or replace it with a better version.

The important thing is to develop a sequence that will enable you to be ready to start, run, and finish the race doing the best possible personal record.

Tip number 39: Always warm up properly before training.

As I said before in other books and articles, I learned the hard way the usefulness of proper warming up. Our tendons, ligaments, and muscles need to warm-up before asking them to produce work and energy.

That's why I stressed in the previous tip that you be at the race start at least an hour before so you will have adequate time to properly warm up your body and prepare it for the running that will start soon.

The way I warm up on races is the same way I warm up while I am training. It's the same set of exercises both in repetitions and duration so doing them on race day it comes out completely naturally, and I do not stress my body with something new. That's why I avoid the warm-up routines the organizers of many races ask from the runners to do because they are doing something completely different of what I trained my body to do. There are two dangers on participating in something new, first, you add to your body stress (physiological) that you can live without, and second, you can injure yourself trying to do exercises that again you did not acclimatize and trained your body to do, risking losing your participation and throw all those months of hard work down the drain. Always have a backup plan like I mentioned earlier.

Tip number 40: Always perform a proper cool down after the race.

I also learned the hard way not to completely stop after the race. It's important to keep moving for at least another 10 to 15 minutes, so you give the chance your muscles to cool down in the movement they were doing the last 2 to 4 hours depending on your distance.

In my first race of 21km when I finished instead of keep moving and walking for a few minutes, I went and sat on a chair and stayed there for 30 minutes. After I had felt that I got some rest, I attempted to get up, and it was, oh my goodness, all the muscles of my body had gotten sore, and I couldn't move at all! I had to ask other people to help me walk to make my muscles start working again!

I repeat, do not stop after the race, the best cool-down you can do is just walk until your heart rate returns to your normal rate. While you walk you can have your water, your electrolytes, some fruit like banana and orange but keep moving until you cool down properly.

Tip number 41: Always simulate the race conditions in training.

It's logical like *Spock* would say, that if your race is going to be in a cold climate, it will be in your best interest to train in a cold climate.

You are not going to train in a hot climate while your race will be in a cold climate and vice versa. The reason you want to have the same or similar weather conditions in training as on race day is twofold. First, you need to acclimatize your body to the weather conditions, achieving the best running economy on the race day.

Second, you will not shock and stress your body on the race day. You will train it with the specific weather conditions, and it will be ready to produce the energy output that was prepared for, achieving the personal records you set as goals.

To give you a very naive example to understand the significance of training in similar weather conditions as the race day, just imagine that you have a chemistry test and instead of reading chemistry exercises, you are reading physics. I hope the analogy made the importance clear.

Tip number 42: Be ready for the unexpected.

Nobody is ever going to be ready for the unexpected, but we can increase our possibilities of being ready to face unexpected problems or situations if we apply ourselves and follow a training program that will enable us to increase our chances of facing and dealing unexpected scenarios with the highest possible success.

Having trained properly, knowing which exercises are working for us and which aren't. Knowing nutrition-wise what food is good for us and which isn't, packing the right stuff for the race, having rituals before the race and on the race day. Having a backup plan; all these will help us deal unexpected events with bigger and better effectiveness.

Have a happy and healthy day.

Andreas Michaelides

www.ingramcontent.com/pod-product-compliance
Lightning Source LLC
Chambersburg PA
CBHW071032280326
41935CB00011B/1542